COLOR THERAPY

A Comprehensive Guide To Explore The Vibrant World Of Emotional Wellness, Energy Balance, And Holistic Healing Through The Language Of Colors

WILFREDO CARSON

INTRODUCTION _________________________________3

CHAPTER 1 _________________________________ *15*

UNDERSTANDING COLOR _________________15

CHAPTER 2 _________________________________ *26*

A HISTORICAL OVERVIEW OF COLOR THERAPY
_________________________________26

CHAPTER 3 _________________________________ *33*

PRINCIPLES OF CHROMATOGRAPHY _______33

CHAPTER 4 _________________________________ *39*

COLORS AND MEANINGS _______________39

CHAPTER 5 _________________________________ *46*

USE OF CHROMOTHERAPY _______________46

CHAPTER 6 _________________________________ *55*

PRACTICAL TECHNIQUES AND EXERCISES __55

CHAPTER 7 _________________________________ *62*

RESEARCH AND CONTROVERSIES _________62

CONCLUSION _________________________________67

INTRODUCTION

Color therapy, also known as chromotherapy, is a holistic approach to healing that uses the vibrational frequencies of colors to promote physical, emotional, and mental health. Color Therapy, which has its roots in ancient civilizations and numerous cultural customs, has grown in favor of modern alternative medicine as a non-invasive and natural approach to a variety of health conditions.

This introduction will provide an explanation of Color Therapy's background, purpose, and breadth, as well as a guide on how to effectively incorporate it into one's life.

1.1 Background on Color Therapy

Color Therapy originated in ancient Egyptian, Chinese, and Indian cultures, where it was believed that various hues held distinct powers and could impact the body's energy centers, or chakras. Ancient Egyptian temples were built with colored glass to harness sunlight's medicinal effects, while color-based remedies were used in Ayurvedic medicine in India. Proponents of color therapy, such as Edwin Babbitt and Dinshah P. Ghadiali, built organized systems in the early twentieth century, which helped to integrate them into Western holistic treatment approaches. Understanding the history of Color Therapy allows us to appreciate its progress and varied cultural influences.

1.2 The purpose and scope of the book

The goal of this book is to provide a full overview of Color Therapy, including its concepts, uses, and potential advantages.

Readers will learn about the psychological and physiological impacts of various colors, as well as practical tips for implementing color therapy into their daily lives. The book's breadth goes beyond theoretical principles to include practical exercises, case studies, and real-life applications, making it an invaluable resource for both beginners and practitioners looking to gain a better grasp of Color Therapy. The book's goal is to empower readers to harness the healing potential of colors for their general well-being by revealing its numerous facets.

1.3 How to Use This Guide.

This handbook is organized in an easy-to-use format to make the knowledge accessible and useful. Each part digs into distinct aspects of Color Therapy, beginning with fundamental ideas and proceeding to more sophisticated topics. Readers are urged to follow the chapter order for complete comprehension, however, each subject can be explored independently for individuals seeking specific information. Practical exercises, case studies, and visuals are used to enrich the learning experience, ensuring a fair mix of theory and practice. As readers progress through the course, they will discover the adaptability of Color Therapy and its ability to be smoothly blended into a variety of lifestyles.

Colour's Psychological Impact

Colour's therapeutic value stems from its psychological impact on human emotions and behaviors. Different hues elicit distinct emotional responses, which influence mood, perception, and general well-being.

Understanding the psychological intricacies of colors is critical for successfully using Color Therapy in a variety of settings.

<u>Color association and symbolism</u>

Colors have cultural, historical, and personal connotations, which add to their symbolic value. Red, for example, is frequently connected with passion and intensity, whilst blue is associated with peace and tranquility. This section delves into the rich network of color connections and symbolism, offering insight into the cultural and individual differences that influence our perceptions of various hues. Understanding these relationships allows practitioners to design color therapy programs to meet the specific needs and preferences of individuals.

Color Psychology and Mind-Body Connection

Color Psychology examines how colors affect the human mind and body. Colors regulate physiological processes in a variety of ways, including increasing neurotransmitter release and altering hormone balance. This section investigates the mind-body relationship in Color Therapy, looking at how specific colors can be deliberately used to treat psychological conditions like stress, anxiety, and depression. By understanding the complex relationship between color and psychology, practitioners can create customized interventions to increase mental and emotional well-being.

Chakras and Energy Centres

The notion of chakras, which is integrated into many holistic systems, recognizes unique energy centers within the body, each of which is connected with a specific hue. Color

Therapy follows chakra concepts by using colors to balance and harmonize these energy centers. This section delves into the relationship between colors and chakras, explaining how practitioners can use Color Therapy to increase energy flow, balance, and general vitality. Understanding the chakra system allows individuals to personalize color therapy practices to specific physical and emotional disorders.

Color Therapy Applications

Color therapy has uses in a variety of settings, including personal well-being practices and therapeutic therapies. This section delves into the various uses of Color Therapy, highlighting its adaptability and usefulness in a variety of settings.

Home and Interior Design

Colors in our living spaces can have a big impact on our mood and energy levels. Color Therapy can be applied in a variety of ways, including home and interior design, which allows people to create spaces that promote health. This section looks into the fundamentals of color in interior design, providing practical advice on choosing and combining colors to improve many elements of life, such as relaxation, focus, and creativity. Individuals can create spaces that promote their overall health by applying color therapy principles to their homes.

<u>Clothing and Personal Style</u>

The colors we wear can influence not only how we see ourselves, but also how others see us. Color Therapy extends to personal style decisions, with certain colors associated with confidence, peacefulness, or brightness. This section investigates the psychological impact of clothing colors and offers tips for adopting Color Therapy to improve personal style. Individuals can use color to express themselves and gain empowerment by aligning their wardrobe choices with certain aims.

<u>Clinical and Therapeutic Settings</u>

Color Therapy has made its way into clinical and therapeutic settings as a complement to traditional treatments. This section investigates the incorporation of Color Therapy into psychotherapy, rehabilitation, and other therapeutic methods. Case examples and research data are offered to demonstrate the potential benefits of color therapy in various clinical settings.

Recognizing its position as a complementary intervention allows practitioners to investigate the synergies between Color Therapy and established therapeutic techniques, thus contributing to holistic and individualized patient treatment.

<u>Art and Creativity</u>

The creative process is inextricably linked with emotions and self-expression. Color plays an important role in artistic pursuits, and this section looks at how Color Therapy can be used to boost creativity and emotional expression through painting. Individuals can utilize color to explore and express their inner ideas and emotions in a variety of artistic disciplines, such as painting and drawing. Individuals who use Color Therapy in their artistic practices can tap into the therapeutic potential of creation as a means of self-discovery and emotional release.

Color therapy, also known as chromotherapy, is a holistic and diverse method of enhancing well-being that uses color vibrational frequencies. Color Therapy, which has its roots in ancient traditions and evolved via many cultural influences, has emerged as a key part of modern alternative medicine. This guide has looked at the history, purpose, and scope of Color Therapy, providing a thorough review for those looking to learn and incorporate this discipline into their life.

Color Therapy covers a wide range of topics, including the psychological impact of colors and their connections, the mind-body link, and chakra alignment. Understanding the relationship between color and psychology enables practitioners to adapt interventions for specific mental and emotional difficulties.

The guide also highlights a variety of Color Therapy uses, including home and interior design, personal style, therapeutic settings, and artistic efforts.

This guide tries to bridge the gap between theory and practice by including practical activities, case studies, and pictures, making Color Therapy accessible to both new and seasoned practitioners. As people investigate the potential of Color Therapy in various aspects of their lives, they can improve their general well-being, stimulate self-expression, and contribute to a more balanced and harmonious existence.

CHAPTER 1
UNDERSTANDING COLOR

The Science of Color

Color therapy, also known as chromotherapy, is based on the fundamental premise that color is a manifestation of light. Color science dives into the electromagnetic spectrum, where visible light accounts for only a small fraction. The Color Spectrum, a range of wavelengths, is essential for understanding the diversity of colors. It ranges from shorter wavelengths such as violet and blue to longer ones like red and orange. This spectrum serves as the foundation for the principles of color therapy.

Color properties include hue, saturation, and brightness.

To navigate the complexities of color therapy, one must first understand color qualities such as hue, saturation, and brightness. Hue refers to a certain color on the spectrum, such as red, green, or any other. Saturation is a measure of a color's intensity or vividness, which ranges from pure to drab. Brightness, on the other hand, refers to the amount of light present, indicating whether a hue appears light or dark. These qualities are important in color therapy because they influence how different colors affect people.

Color Perception

Human Eye and Color Vision

Understanding color therapy involves knowledge of human color perception. The human eye is a marvel of biological ingenuity, capable of seeing a wide range of colors.

The retina of the eye contains photoreceptor cells known as cones and rods, which are important for color vision. Color perception is possible thanks to cones, which are sensitive to different wavelengths. The brain processes messages from these cones, resulting in the beautiful tapestry of colors that people see. This complicated process is the foundation for how color therapy interacts with the human visual system.

Cultural and Psychological Influences

The psychological and cultural aspects of color perception are critical to the efficacy of color therapy. Colors have particular meanings in different cultures around the world, and these cultural connotations influence how people react to them. Furthermore, psychological aspects such as emotions, memories, and personal experiences influence how people respond to particular hues. Understanding these variables is critical for adapting color therapy interventions to people and comprehending the complex interplay of biology, culture, and psychology.

<u>Application of Color Therapy</u>

Color Therapy for Healing.

Color therapy has gained popularity as a holistic method of healing. Different colors are said to have distinct energy qualities that can affect physical, emotional, and mental health. For example, warm colors like red and orange are associated with stimulation and activity, but cold colors like blue and green are associated with relaxation and peace. Color therapists utilize specific colors to address various disorders or imbalances in the body, restore harmony, and improve general health.

Chakra and Color Therapy

Color therapy and the concept of chakras are frequently linked to alternative medical and spiritual traditions. Chakras are energy centers in the body that are each connected with a distinct color. The alignment of these energy centers is regarded as critical for preserving bodily and mental balance. Color therapy is used to balance and align the chakras, with practitioners using specific colors for each chakra to aid healing and regulate energy flow throughout the body.

Color Therapy in Psychology.

Color therapy is based on the psychological impact of colors. Various colors are thought to elicit distinct feelings and moods.

For example, yellow is connected with positivity and enthusiasm, whereas purple may represent reflection and spiritual progress. Psychologists and therapists use color therapy in their work to create surroundings that promote emotional well-being or elicit certain responses from patients. This interdisciplinary approach acknowledges the fundamental relationship between color, emotion, and psychological states.

<u>Color Therapy for Design and Aesthetics</u>

Beyond healing and psychology, color therapy is expressed through design and aesthetics. Color theory investigates how different colors combine to create harmony or contrast. Designers use the emotional and psychological influence of colors to elicit various reactions in people.

 Color selections are purposefully chosen to impact perceptions, attitudes, and behaviors in anything from advertising to interior design. Understanding color theory is, therefore, necessary for workers in domains where aesthetics and visual impact are important.

<u>Critiques and controversies</u>

Scientific skepticism

Despite its popularity, color therapy is viewed skeptically by the scientific community.

The absence of scientific evidence to support color therapy's therapeutic claims calls into doubt its efficacy. Skeptics claim that the subjective nature of color perception, as well as the lack of established techniques, make it difficult to develop a solid scientific foundation for color therapy. This criticism emphasizes the importance of doing comprehensive research to support or invalidate the therapeutic claims related to color therapy.

<u>Cultural variability and appropriation</u>

The cultural dimension of color therapy creates issues in terms of variety and appropriation. Colors have various connotations throughout cultures, and what is considered therapeutic in one culture may be improper or even harmful in another. Color therapists must manage cultural variety with caution, understanding the possibility of misinterpretation or appropriation. Furthermore, the commercialization of color therapy products and activities creates ethical difficulties because cultural symbols and rituals risk becoming commodities for mass consumption.

Individual Variability and Subjectivity

Another criticism levelled toward color therapy is the individual variety and subjective nature of color perception. Colors can elicit various feelings and behaviors depending on personal experiences, memories, and psychological states. Some color therapy approaches take a one-size-fits-all approach that may not appropriately meet individuals' distinct needs and sensitivities. Color therapy methods must be tailored to account for individual heterogeneity and subjectivity to improve their therapeutic efficacy.

Color therapy, often known as chromotherapy, is a multifaceted method that incorporates color science, human perception, and cultural influences. Understanding the color spectrum, color characteristics, and the complexities of human color vision lays the groundwork for investigating the therapeutic applications of color.

The psychological and cultural components of color perception add to the field's richness, emphasizing the intricate interplay of biology, culture, and psychology in shaping individual color responses.

Color therapy has a wide range of applications, including health, psychology, design, and aesthetics. Its use in alternative medicine, especially in connection with chakras, emphasizes the holistic aspect of this approach. However, color therapy is not without its difficulties, including scientific skepticism, worries about cultural variety and appropriation, and the need to address individual variation and subjectivity.

As color therapy evolves, robust scientific research and ethical issues will be critical to establishing its legitimacy and responsible application. Balancing color therapy's artistic, cultural, and therapeutic features can help it become more widely adopted, providing individuals with a potentially helpful and holistic approach to improving well-being.

CHAPTER 2
A HISTORICAL OVERVIEW OF COLOR THERAPY

Color therapy, often known as chromotherapy, has a long history that includes numerous ancient cultures. In terms of ancient techniques, Ayurveda, India's traditional medical system, was significant in bringing color therapy into its holistic approach. Ayurveda believes in harmonizing the body's doshas (Vata, Pitta, and Kapha), and color therapy was used to achieve this equilibrium. Each color was connected with particular therapeutic properties that affected both physical and mental health. The use of colors in Ayurveda extends back thousands of years, demonstrating the profound relationship between hue and health.

pg. 26

Similarly, Chinese medicine, which has its roots in ancient philosophy, included the concept of color in its healing methods. The ancient Chinese believed in the balance of Yin and Yang, as well as the Five Elements theory, which linked colors to various elements and organ systems. Color therapy was utilized to balance the body's energy flow (Qi) and preserve harmony. The use of color in Chinese medicine demonstrates an early knowledge of the powerful impact color can have on the human body, which predates modern scientific understanding.

The Impact of Color on Western Traditions

Color therapy has had an impact on Western cultures since the Middle Ages and Renaissance. During these periods, the concept of sympathetic magic was popular, and colors were thought to have special vibrations that might alter the natural world. This notion provided the foundation for using colors in numerous healing procedures. In medieval Europe, stained glass windows in cathedrals were not only renowned for their aesthetic appeal but also for their healing abilities, with each color signifying a particular aspect of spiritual and physical healing.

The Renaissance period enhanced our understanding of color therapy. Visionaries such as Paracelsus and Leonardo da Vinci investigated the relationship between color, light, and health.

Paracelsus, a Swiss physician, alchemist, and astrologer, believed that colors had curative properties and were associated with fluid balance in the body.

Leonardo da Vinci's studies in optics and color theory contributed to our growing understanding of how colors influence human perception and well-being.

Modern Development of Chromotherapy

The current evolution of chromotherapy gained traction in the nineteenth and twentieth centuries, owing to scientific developments and an increased interest in alternative medical approaches. Early pioneers, such as Dinshah P. Ghadiali, contributed significantly to the formalization of chromotherapy.

Ghadiali, an Indian-American scientist, created the Spectro-Chrome method, which entailed exposing patients to certain hues of light to treat a variety of health conditions. His study paved the way for the systematic use of color therapy in the clinical context.

As scientific expertise grew, experts investigated the physiological and psychological effects of colors on the human body. Researchers began to investigate how different colors affected mood, emotions, and overall well-being.

The birth of color psychology, a subject that studies the psychological impacts of color, helped to bridge the gap between old traditions and modern scientific study. Color therapy, which was formerly considered mystical or esoteric, has begun to acquire respect as a complementary technique within traditional medicine.

Chromotherapy now has applications in a variety of sectors, including holistic medicine, psychology, and design. Color therapy is frequently used in integrative healthcare settings to complement conventional treatments and improve the overall healing experience. The use of color in architecture and interior design demonstrates an understanding of how the color palette of the environment affects occupants' moods and productivity. The evolution of chromotherapy from ancient traditions to modern applications demonstrates the enduring curiosity and recognition of color's capacity to promote well-being.

The history of color therapy demonstrates an intriguing progression from ancient techniques centered in Ayurveda and Chinese medicine to the pivotal eras of medieval and Renaissance Europe.

The modern evolution of chromotherapy, fueled by scientific research and pioneers such as Dinshah P. Ghadiali, has elevated color therapy to a recognized and integrated area within healthcare and design. Color's continuing relevance in promoting holistic well-being demonstrates its varied impact on the human experience.

CHAPTER 3
PRINCIPLES OF CHROMATOGRAPHY

Chromotherapy, also known as color therapy, is a holistic treatment approach that stretches back to ancient civilizations. It is based on the notion that colors may have a profound impact on the human body, mind, and soul. The ideas of chromotherapy are based on the idea that different hues have particular vibrational frequencies and that exposure to specific colors can affect many aspects of our well-being. These concepts are based on the understanding that the human body is made up of energy and that colors can help restore balance and improve overall health.

Chromotherapy in Healing.

Chromotherapy is widely utilized as a treatment modality to address physical, emotional, and spiritual problems. The main principle is to use colors to stimulate the body's energy centers, commonly known as chakras. Each chakra is connected with a certain color, and using these hues is said to restore balance to the accompanying energy center. Color therapy practitioners aim to establish a balanced flow of energy throughout the body by aligning the chakras, hence helping the natural healing process.

Balancing energy centers (chakras)

Chromotherapy is based on the concept of balancing energy centers, or chakras. Traditional Eastern philosophies consider these energy centers to be essential components of the body's energy system. Each chakra is connected with a certain organ, emotion, or facet of consciousness. Chromotherapy gives certain hues to each chakra, with the hope that exposure to these colors will bring about balance and healing. For example, the root chakra, associated with the color red, is said to govern issues of survival and grounding, whereas the crown chakra, associated with violet or white, is associated with spiritual awareness.

Aura and Color

Chromotherapy's influence extends beyond the physical body to the subtle energy field known as the aura. The aura is thought to represent one's overall well-being and can be changed by exposure to different hues. Chronotherapies believe that specific colors help cleanse, strengthen, or protect the aura, resulting in a better energy field. Understanding the interaction of colors and auras is important in the holistic approach of chromotherapy because it tackles not only the physical elements of health but also the energetic and spiritual dimensions.

<u>Color and Mind</u>

Colors are believed to have a tremendous effect on the mind, impacting emotions, ideas, and cognitive functions. Chromotherapy recognizes the complex relationship between color and the mind and uses this relationship for therapeutic reasons.

Emotional Responses to Color

Chromotherapy investigates the psychological effect of colors on human emotions. Different colors are thought to elicit specific emotional responses, and practitioners employ this information to design therapeutic spaces. Warm tones, such as red and orange, are connected with energy, passion, and warmth, whereas cool tones, such as blue and green, represent calmness and tranquillity. Chromotherapy attempts to improve emotional states and mental health by deliberately combining various hues into healing places.

<u>Color and Cognitive Function</u>

Colors have an impact on both emotions and cognitive abilities. Chromotherapy investigates how different colors can stimulate or relax the mind, increase concentration, and even improve memory. According to several research, exposure to specific colors of blue may improve mental attention and productivity.

Chronotherapies use this information to construct surroundings that promote cognitive well-being, taking into account aspects such as color intensity, brightness, and hue to achieve optimal conditions for mental clarity and performance.

Chromotherapy is a holistic method of healing that integrates energy balance, emotional well-being, and cognitive performance. The use of color in this holistic therapy reflects an old idea that is still relevant in modern holistic therapies, providing a unique viewpoint on the interdependence of the body, mind, and spirit.

CHAPTER 4
COLORS AND MEANINGS

Color therapy, also known as chromotherapy, is a comprehensive strategy that uses colors to improve physical, emotional, and mental health. Each color is said to have distinct energy and psychological impacts on people. In this thorough investigation, we dive into the meanings and therapeutic effects of many hues, providing light on the enormous impact they may have on human physiology and mind.

<u>Red: The Energizer.</u>

Red, which is typically connected with passion and intensity, is regarded as the energizer in color therapy. It is thought to stimulate and boost energy levels, making it an excellent choice for anybody experiencing exhaustion or lethargy. In chromotherapy, red is related to the root chakra, which represents stability and energy. It is thought to improve blood circulation, elevate heart rate, and increase general physical vitality. However, excessive exposure to red can cause restlessness or heightened emotions, emphasizing the careful balance required when adding red to therapeutic techniques.

Orange: The Creativity Booster.

Orange is connected with warmth, excitement, and inventiveness in chromotherapy. Orange is said to inspire creative thinking and foster a sense of joy. It is commonly used to stimulate the mind and boost the soul. In terms of chakras, orange corresponds to the sacral chakra, which controls emotions and creativity. Incorporating orange into one's environment or attire is thought to promote self-expression and artistic endeavors. However, like with any color, balance is essential, since excessive exposure to orange may result in overstimulation.

<u>Yellow: the Optimizer</u>

Yellow, which is associated with sunlight and cheerfulness, is considered the optimizer in chromotherapy. This color is thought to improve mental clarity, increase intellectual activities, and boost optimism.

Yellow is commonly associated with the solar plexus chakra, which represents personal power and self-esteem. Yellow is supposed to increase confidence and promote an optimistic mentality. However, caution should be exercised because continuous exposure to bright yellow may cause uneasiness or nervousness.

Green: the balancer.

Green, which represents nature and balance, serves as a balancing color in color therapy.

It is connected with peace, development, and renewal. Green is frequently used to promote a sense of balance and serenity, making it an excellent choice for stress reduction.

Green corresponds to the heart chakra, which represents love and compassion. This color is thought to have a calming impact on both the mind and the body, encouraging emotional well-being. However, incorrect use or exposure to specific shades of green can cause feelings of stagnation or dullness.

Blue: The Calmer.

Blue, which is frequently associated with tranquility and serenity, serves as a calming agent in chromotherapy. It is thought to have a significant effect in reducing stress and anxiety and promoting relaxation. Blue is related to the throat chakra, which represents speech and self-expression. The use of blue in the environment is supposed to promote open communication and clarity of mind. However, it is critical to achieve a balance, as excessive exposure to particular shades of blue can cause emotions of sadness or solitude.

<u>Indigo: The intuitive</u>

Indigo, a deep and enigmatic color, is considered intuitive in color therapy. It is related to spiritual consciousness and increased intuition. The indigo color is generally associated with the third eye chakra, which controls insight and intuition.

Indigo is said to provide a greater understanding of oneself and the spiritual realm. It is regarded as an effective instrument for meditation and introspection. Individuals should approach indigo with caution, since excessive use may result in emotions of detachment or hypersensitivity.

<u>Violet, The Spiritual Enhancer</u>

Violet, the color of spirituality and enlightenment, acts as a spiritual booster in chromotherapy. Violet is associated with the crown chakra, which signifies higher consciousness and is thought to help people connect with their spiritual selves. It is frequently used to help people meditate, find inner peace, and progress spiritually.

However, it is critical to exercise caution because extended exposure to bright violet may cause emotions of escapism or separation from the physical world.

The notions of color therapy dive deeply into the psychological and physiological effects of colors on human health. Understanding the meanings and therapeutic effects of each color enables people to take advantage of chromotherapy's potential benefits in creating balance, harmony, and overall well-being. As with any holistic approach, moderation and individual sensitivity should be addressed to ensure that the use of color is appropriate for each individual seeking therapeutic benefits.

CHAPTER 5
USE OF CHROMOTHERAPY

Color has a major impact on many elements of human existence, including not only our visual perceptions but also our emotions, moods, and overall well-being. Chromotherapy, often known as color therapy, is a holistic method that uses colors to promote physical, mental, and emotional well-being. This therapeutic technique has found applications in a wide range of sectors, including interior design, alternative medicine, and even beauty and fashion.

<u>Color in Interior Design.</u>

Color is extremely important in interior design since it has a significant impact on the atmosphere and aesthetics of a room.

Designers frequently utilize color intentionally to create a unified and visually pleasing atmosphere. Choosing colors for living spaces necessitates careful consideration of the psychological and emotional effects that each color can have on people. Warm colors, such as reds and yellows, may generate feelings of vitality and warmth, whilst cool colors, such as blues and greens, can encourage a sense of serenity and tranquillity. The choosing of colors in interior design is more than just personal taste; it also requires a grasp of color psychology and its impact on occupants.

<u>Color Theory for Interior Design</u>

Color psychology is an important part of interior design that studies people's emotional and psychological responses to various hues.

pg. 47

The use of color psychology in home decor can be seen in the hues chosen for different spaces. To improve relaxation and sleep quality, bedrooms can be painted in relaxing colors such as gentle blues or greens. Living rooms, on the other hand, may use more brilliant hues, such as oranges or yellows, to encourage conversation and connection. Understanding the emotional influence of colors enables designers to create rooms that meet specific demands, promoting a balance between aesthetics and utility in domestic designs.

<u>Chromotherapy in Alternative Medicine.</u>

Chromotherapy has spread its influence to alternative medicine, where the therapeutic use of colors is said to enhance the body's natural healing processes. Light therapy, a crucial component of chromotherapy, entails exposing people to certain colors or wavelengths of light to treat a variety of physical and mental health concerns. Different colors have distinct healing qualities.

For example, red light is said to increase circulation and activity, but blue light is commonly employed for its relaxing benefits. This strategy is based on the belief that colors can impact the body's energy centers, known as chakras, to restore balance and harmony.

<u>Light Therapy</u>

Light therapy, a type of chromotherapy, is the regulated exposure of patients to specific wavelengths of light to address a variety of health conditions. This therapy method has acquired popularity in the treatment of seasonal affective disorder (SAD), sleeplessness, and some skin ailments.

For example, exposure to bright white light is frequently utilized to treat SAD symptoms by simulating natural sunlight. The wavelengths of light utilized in treatment sessions are carefully chosen for their ability to influence the body's circadian rhythm and hormonal balance, demonstrating the complex relationship between color and physiological well-being.

Color Meditation

Color meditation is another alternative health approach that uses chromotherapy principles. Focusing on a certain hue or a sequence of colors during meditation promotes relaxation, balance, and emotional well-being. Practitioners believe that each color correlates to a specific energy center in the body and that meditating on these colors can help people restore equilibrium to these energy centers. For example, envisioning a tranquil blue light during meditation may be intended to promote calmness and reduce tension. Color meditation is a holistic technique for gaining mental clarity and emotional balance by utilizing the healing power of various hues.

Colors in Beauty and Fashion

The impact of chromotherapy extends beyond interior design and alternative treatment to beauty and fashion. The idea that colors can influence emotions and well-being has led to the incorporation of color therapy ideas into people's clothing, accessories, and even makeup selections.

<u>Wearing Colors for Wellbeing.</u>

Choosing clothing based on color for well-being is a technique that supports the notion that colors can influence an individual's mood and energy levels. Someone looking for an energy boost, for example, may choose apparel in bright, warm colors such as red or orange. Someone who wants to feel peaceful and balanced, on the other hand, may dress in soothing colors like blue or green.

The use of chromotherapy in fashion is not only a personal style choice, but also a purposeful decision to improve one's emotional condition by intentionally selecting colors that correspond to various feelings and energies.

Makeup and Color Therapy

The relationship between makeup and color therapy is especially visible in the beauty business, where makeup color selection extends beyond aesthetics to influence the wearer's emotional condition. Colors can influence perceptions and moods; which makeup artists and aficionados understand. Warm-toned cosmetics tones, such as reds and oranges, can represent passion and confidence, whilst cool-toned shades, such as blues and purples, can suggest calm and sophistication. The intentional use of colors in makeup application demonstrates a grasp of how chromotherapy concepts can be applied not just to visual enhancement but also to persons' psychological and emotional well-being.

Chromotherapy has a wide range of uses, including interior design, alternative

pg. 53

medicine, cosmetics, and fashion. The deep relationship between colors and human emotions serves as the foundation for chromotherapy, which involves the intentional use of specific hues to improve physical, mental, and emotional equilibrium. Whether used in the selection of paint for living spaces, light therapy in alternative medicine, or the selection of clothing and makeup in beauty and fashion, chromotherapy continues to captivate people seeking a holistic approach to well-being through the therapeutic power of colors.

CHAPTER 6
PRACTICAL TECHNIQUES AND EXERCISES

Color therapy, also known as chromotherapy, is a holistic healing technique that uses the vibrational frequencies of colors to promote physical, emotional, and mental health.

This therapeutic technique is based on the idea that different colors have unique energy signatures that might affect many aspects of a person's health. Several essential themes stand out among the practical procedures and exercises used in Color Therapy: color breathing, color visualization, color bathing, color meditation practices, and color incorporation into daily life.

Color Breathing is a fundamental method in Color Therapy that emphasizes the deliberate inhaling and exhalation of specific hues to balance and align the body's energy centers. Practitioners frequently equate different colors with specific chakras, which are energy centers within the body according to traditional Eastern philosophies. For example, red may represent the root chakra, whereas blue may represent the throat chakra. Practitioners visualize inhaling a specific color to absorb its energy properties and eliminate any imbalances or obstructions. This technique not only promotes relaxation but also aims to improve an individual's overall vitality by balancing energy flow within the body.

Color Visualization is another important part of Color Therapy that involves using conscious mental imaging of specific colors to achieve desired results.

This practice explores the psychological and emotional responses connected with various hues. Warm tones, such as red and orange, are frequently connected with greater energy and vigor, whilst cooler tones, such as blue and green, can be associated with relaxation and tranquillity. Color Visualization is used in guided meditation sessions, when people are urged to concentrate their minds on a certain color, allowing its healing effects to materialize in their thoughts and feelings. This technique is especially effective for reducing stress, restoring emotional equilibrium, and encouraging a positive attitude.

Color Bathing is a relaxing and immersive Color Therapy activity that entails surrounding oneself with a certain color, usually through the use of colored lighting or bath additives. This approach is inspired by the ancient practice of chromotherapy baths, in which people would immerse themselves in water laced with natural hues. Modern Color Therapy uses colored lights or bath salts to provide a regulated and adjustable experience. Each hue is thought to have unique healing effects, and people can select colors based on their therapeutic aims. For example, a red bath may be chosen for its stimulating and invigorating benefits, whereas a blue bath is chosen for its relaxation and stress-reduction properties.

Color Meditation Practices go beyond basic imagery by adopting a deeper meditative approach to harnessing the therapeutic advantages of colors.

Color meditation allows people to focus on a single color or proceed through a series of colors to accomplish certain results.

This practice frequently incorporates mindfulness techniques, in which practitioners build present-moment awareness while immersing themselves in the vibrational energy of the chosen color. Color Meditation Practices are intended to increase self-awareness, promote mental clarity, and foster a sense of balance and harmony among individuals.

This approach is generally embraced for its ability to reduce anxiety, improve focus, and promote overall mental health.

Incorporating Colors into Daily Life is a comprehensive method of Color Therapy that encourages people to include certain colors in their daily environments, activities, and decisions. This approach acknowledges that the power of colors extends beyond targeted therapeutic sessions and pervades many parts of one's life. This could include selecting clothing in specific colors to elicit desired moods or energy, decorating living spaces with colors that promote relaxation or creativity, or even selecting foods with brilliant hues said to have special health benefits. Individuals who actively incorporate colors into their everyday lives hope to create an atmosphere that consistently supports their well-being, developing a harmonic interaction between the individual and the energetic properties of various colors.

The practical strategies and activities in Color Therapy provide a varied range of ways to promote overall well-being. Color Breathing, Color Visualization, Color Bathing, Color Meditation Practices, and Using Colors in Daily Life give people a variety of methods for dealing with physical, emotional, and mental health issues. These techniques combine ancient wisdom, psychological principles, and vibrational energy concepts to provide a comprehensive framework for individuals looking to explore the healing power of colors systematically and deliberately. As Color Therapy gains popularity in the field of complementary and alternative medicine, further research and investigation into its efficacy and mechanisms may shed light on the complex relationship between color and human well-being.

CHAPTER 7
RESEARCH AND CONTROVERSIES

Chromotherapy, often known as color therapy, is a holistic treatment approach based on the notion that certain hues can affect many elements of human health and well-being. Chromotherapy research has sought to elucidate the underlying mechanics and efficacy of this alternative treatment. Researchers studied how different colors affect physiological processes like heart rate, blood pressure, and hormone levels. Researchers have also investigated the psychological and emotional effects of color on humans, attempting to discover links between color perception and mental states.

While some studies imply that chromotherapy may have benefits, the discipline is not without controversy. Critics believe that the scientific evidence for color therapy's therapeutic claims is frequently inconclusive and lacking in rigorous experimental design. Furthermore, the subjective character of individual color reactions makes it difficult to standardize experimental techniques. The dependence on anecdotal evidence, as well as the lack of large-scale, well-controlled clinical research, add to the skepticism about chromotherapy. As the scientific community grapples with these concerns, the current study helps us better grasp the potential mechanisms underlying color's effects on the human body and mind.

Criticism and Skepticism:

Critics and skeptics of chromotherapy point to a lack of a strong scientific foundation and a dependence on anecdotal data to back up its claims. Skeptics believe that the apparent therapeutic effects of specific colors could be due to a placebo reaction or psychological factors rather than a direct physiological influence. Furthermore, the lack of a defined method for color therapy treatments, as well as the vast range of techniques among practitioners, raises concerns about its legitimacy.

Furthermore, some critics are concerned about the commercialization of color therapy goods without adequate scientific support. The promotion of color therapy as a cure-all for a variety of ailments, without strong empirical evidence, raises ethical concerns. Skeptics stress the necessity of distinguishing between pseudoscientific claims and evidence-based procedures to safeguard consumers from potentially misleading information.

Addressing these issues will necessitate a collaborative effort among the scientific community to produce well-designed, controlled research that can objectively quantify the impact of color on health outcomes. This includes looking into the potential placebo effects of chromotherapy and determining whether any true physiological mechanisms are at play.

Future Trends and Development:

Despite the criticism and controversies surrounding chromotherapy, recent trends and advancements indicate a growing interest in researching its possible applications. Researchers are increasingly turning to interdisciplinary techniques, combining findings from psychology, neurology, and traditional medicine to develop a better understanding of how color affects human health.

Technological advancements, such as neuroimaging tools, provide new opportunities to investigate the neurological correlates of color perception and its effects on the brain. These cutting-edge techniques may aid in unraveling the complexities of the mind-body link involved with chromotherapy. Furthermore, collaborations between researchers and practitioners in the field may result in the creation of established protocols and standards for the use of color therapy in therapeutic settings.

The incorporation of chromotherapy into mainstream healthcare procedures is a possible future trend, assuming robust scientific studies support its effectiveness.

As the demand for alternative and complementary therapies grows, there is a need for open communication among academics, healthcare providers, and the general public to develop a responsible and evidence-based approach to incorporating chromotherapy into wellness plans.

CONCLUSION

Color therapy, often known as chromotherapy, is still a field marked by both enthusiasm and skepticism. Scientific research has investigated the potential physiological and psychological impacts of exposure to various hues, with some promising results.

However, the lack of established methods, inconsistent methodology, and the subjective nature of individual responses have sparked debate and criticism within the scientific community.

The concerns and skepticism surrounding chromotherapy emphasize the importance of conducting robust research using well-designed, controlled experiments. Addressing these challenges would necessitate collaboration among scientists, practitioners, and policymakers to develop evidence-based practices and recommendations.

As technology progresses, using neuroscientific methods to investigate the neurological underpinnings of color perception may reveal additional insights into chromotherapy's therapeutic potential.

Looking ahead, chromotherapy trends and advancements indicate a shift toward multidisciplinary study and possible inclusion into mainstream healthcare. However, this progress must be accompanied by a commitment to transparency, ethical considerations, and responsible communication to provide the public with accurate information regarding color therapy's benefits and limitations. As the scientific community works to overcome these obstacles, the ultimate goal is to lay a firm foundation for the study and implementation of chromotherapy in improving human well-being.